Pixiwoo

After both finding careers in the make-up industry, sisters Nic and Sam joined together to create the Pixiwoo brand. Their highly successful YouTube makeup channel has over two million subscribers, with each video generating hundreds of thousands of views. Sam and Nic are the faces of the globally famous Real Techniques brush collection. Sam and Nic continue to grow as top artistic consultants, writing columns for national magazines and newspapers, appearing on major network television as beauty experts, and editing their own digital magazine.

PERFECT
SKIN

COMPACT MAKE-UP GUIDE

TOOLS • SKIN • FINISHES

PERFECT
SKIN

COMPACT MAKE-UP GUIDE

TOOLS • SKIN • FINISHES

SAM AND NIC CHAPMAN

Published by Blink Publishing
3.25, The Plaza,
535 Kings Road,
Chelsea Harbour,
London, SW10 0SZ

www.blinkpublishing.co.uk

facebook.com/blinkpublishing
twitter.com/blinkpublishing

Perfect Skin – 978-1-911600-45-9

A CIP catalogue of this book is available from the British Library.

Printed and bound in Lithuania.

1 3 5 7 9 10 8 6 4 2

Text copyright © Samantha Chapman and Nicola Haste/Pixiwoo Limited, 2017
Images © Sam and Nic Chapman, Real Techniques, James Lincoln, Simon Songhurst, Elisabeth Hoff and Shutterstock.
Design by Type & Numbers Creative. www.typeandnumbers.com

Papers used by Blink Publishing are natural, recyclable products made from wood grown in sustainable forests. The manufacturing processes conform to the environmental regulations of the country of origin.

Blink Publishing is an imprint of the Bonnier Publishing Group
www.bonnierpublishing.co.uk

For Mum, without your love and support
none of this would have been possible.

FACE

APP BY

Pixiwoo

THE ULTIMATE MAKE-UP AND BEAUTY GUIDE ON YOUR SCREEN!

Create the perfect look for every occasion with the Face App by Pixiwoo! The dynamic duo, Sam and Nic Chapman, share their extensive beauty knowledge and make-up expertise with exclusive digital content. From never-before-seen video tutorials, pictures and helpful tips to special features such as the Selfie Booth, the Face App by Pixiwoo will help you achieve the incredible looks Sam and Nic are known for.

To access all this exclusive content, download the free app from the iTunes App Store or Google Play Store, launch the app and point your device's camera at the pages with the special phone icon (right) on them. Here all of Pixiwoo's advice and special features will come to life on your screen!

FOR THE ULTIMATE FACE EXPERIENCE DON'T FORGET TO USE YOUR FREE AND UNIQUE PIXIWOO COLOUR WHEEL FOUND IN THE APP'S MAIN MENU

*The Face App by Pixiwoo requires an Internet connection to be downloaded and can be used on iPhone, iPad or Android devices. For direct links to download the app and further information, visit www.blinkpublishing.co.uk

SCAN THIS PAGE NOW FOR YOUR FIRST VIDEO!

CONTENTS

10

INTRODUCTION

24

TOOLS OF THE TRADE

68

SKIN

146

FINISHES

MEET THE
AUTHORS

SAM & NIC

We have been educating women and men of all ages in the art of make-up for over 20 years. We developed Pixiwoo on social media back in 2008.

Pixiwoo was born out of our hard-earned knowledge and passion for make-up and we never imagined it would become our actual career. The success of our channel has enabled us to branch out in many areas.

We have taught hundreds of new make-up artists and we are always inspired by our students' enthusiasm and passion for make-up. We decided to use our knowledge of what people need to learn to produce some easy-to-follow books that break down facial make-up and how to apply it, along with application techniques and our anecdotes and tips.

We wanted to get back to basics and assist beginners or students of the industry and also offer opinions and tips to working make-up artists.

We wanted to also incorporate our social media background and include interactive apps for extra product information, colour theory assistance and brand-new tutorials created especially for you.

You will learn more about us personally, along with our opinions on the best products and also the techniques we normally edit out of our tutorials. You may wonder why we select certain products and tools for our tutorial videos and this book will tell you.

We have loved compiling our knowledge for you and if you are a total make-up beginner and are unsure of where to start then this book will be your companion. If you are just setting out in the industry we will offer you insider tips and advice for your journey.

We hope you enjoy!

SAM

I always knew I wanted to do something involving make-up and creativity. As with most siblings, Nic and I squabbled regularly. Nic was the annoying little sister who enjoyed nothing better than trying to wind me up or embarrass me. The only thing that united us was our love of make-up. We loved to watch our mum apply her own make-up and took a great interest in our auntie's career as a make-up artist.

In 1993, after leaving school, I enrolled in a two-year BTEC course in media make-up before moving to London to assist our aunt. I was excited to get away from rural Norfolk and be independent.

I began working on a make-up counter, which gave me confidence with different skin types and tones. I moved to a make-up studio in London where I created suitable looks while working fast.

After two years I began working for MAC in the Carnaby Street Pro Store and later became part of their Pro Team. I travelled extensively to create high-fashion looks for the various fashion weeks and assisted top make-up artists, including Val Garland, Charlotte Tilbury, Sharon Dowsett and Tom Pecheux. Life was pretty hectic but I was really focused on building up my personal portfolio so I would test with other creatives. I also did freelance work including bridal make-up as I was always conscious of having a back-up plan.

In 2003 I got my first agent and was soon booked for magazines and celebrity shoots. I left MAC and worked part-time for Chanel. A year later I had my first daughter, Lily. I continued to work freelance, including doing the make-up for artists at MTV and teaching at a make-up school.

Shortly before the birth of my second daughter, Olivia, I started the Pixiwoo YouTube channel. Nic's childhood nickname was Pixi and my email address then included the word 'Pixiwoo'. I used the name without thinking about how it would become our brand's logo. We like it, though, and there isn't much else out there similar to it.

My first tutorial created a look for a client who wanted a smoky eye. I felt writing the information wouldn't really give her a feel for it – plus I hated to write – so I filmed it instead. The client loved it and more people started to watch and request looks. It started to get really popular and I couldn't manage the workload. By then Nic and I had grown closer and the time we'd spent apart had made us appreciate each other. Nic was always very supportive and was also working in the industry so I asked her if she would like to join me. For two years we worked solidly on the channel, trying to build its popularity. I created tutorials that worked better with my features while Nic's suited her style and look.

The hard work got us noticed and in 2010 Real Techniques approached us. I became Artistic Consultant initially and helped them create a new, different type of make-up brush that performed exceptionally well at an affordable price. The brush range was based on our growing social media success. In 2013, when Nic was able to devote more energy to the brand, we became joint Artistic Consultants. Real Techniques has gone on to become the most popular make-up brush in the UK. It's also now currently the fastest growing make-up brush brand in the US.

We continue to push our brand and never take any of our opportunities for granted. We have worked so hard to build Pixiwoo and we try and take each day as it comes. We still have our fights and have very different ways of approaching situations but we always pull together and make a great team.

NICOLA

I was never really academic at school. I loved sports and art but as we grew up in rural Norfolk I was more interested in being outdoors with my friends. I had imagined I would be a nurse as I loved caring for people and this seemed like a natural progression for me.

When I eventually left school I still wasn't quite sure what to do next. Our mum's sister, Maggie, is a successful make-up artist and I loved listening to her talk about her glamorous clients and decided that this might be a fun industry to work in. Sam had already gone on to college to study make-up, and she encouraged me to give it a try. I studied a BTEC National Diploma at college and had a great two years but I still needed extra training and guidance. I don't think you ever really learn until you are in the industry.

I assisted my aunt and also gained valuable work experience at Nicky Clarke and Jo Hansford, both premium hairdressers in London. Based on my good work ethic they both offered me a job, but I was focused on make-up.

I returned to Norfolk and landed a job for Estée Lauder working on the counter and gradually worked my way up to counter manager. I heard that there was a MAC store coming to Norwich and working for a sister brand helped me to get an interview.

I was so excited and I can still remember the make-up I wore. A combination of So There Jade and Minted eyeliner, a vibrant green mascara called Boston Fern and a baby pink lipstick called Snob. It was a winning combination and I became an assistant manager.

I remained in this position for four years and made some great friends before becoming a supervisor at the MAC Pro Store in Carnaby Street, London, for three years. I would often freelance in the evenings – bridal work, drag make-up and editorial work. Then I joined Illamasqua in Selfridges.

In 2008 Sam told me that she had started recording make-up tutorials on YouTube and had begun to get lots of requests for looks. She asked if I wanted to help create some tutorials. Sam never really had a massive plan but we decided to create fun and informative content.

I really enjoyed helping her but it was hard working full-time and freelancing too. I decided that I would return home to Norfolk and give this YouTube thing a go! I knew I could always fall back on bridal make-up work. We started creating looks for the channel and at the weekend we worked together as bridal make-up artists to earn some money. This was the first time in years we had been in each other's presence regularly but the time apart had drawn us closer.

I soon met my husband, Ian, and I knew that Norfolk was where I wanted to be so Sam and I focused really hard on the Pixiwoo channel. In 2010 we were approached by Real Techniques to help create a new type of make-up brush. Sadly I had two miscarriages and just needed to focus on myself. I just helped behind the scenes at Real Techniques. Fortunately, Ian and I went on to have two beautiful children, Harry and Edie. I then joined the Real Techniques team with Sam as an Artistic Consultant while creating weekly tutorials for Pixiwoo.

We never like to plan too far ahead and take each day as it comes. We know each other's strengths and also when the other is struggling. Every week brings a new challenge but we deal with it together.

TOOLS

*"The right tools are just as important
as the make-up itself."*

——————————————— *Bobbi Brown*

WHAT TOOLS YOU NEED

DEPENDS ON YOUR CIRCUMSTANCES. A MAKE-UP ARTIST WORKING IN THE INDUSTRY WILL HAVE A DIFFERENT SET OF REQUIREMENTS FROM SOMEONE WHO NEEDS THE FUNDAMENTALS TO GET THEM THROUGH THE DAY. WE'LL TAKE YOU THROUGH SOME GREAT IDEAS SO YOU CAN PICK WHAT WORKS BEST FOR YOU.

BASIC TOOLS

Nobody has one tone to their skin and, although it's unrealistic for everyone to purchase multiple foundations, you can often get the perfect shade by mixing from a variety of colours, just as an artist would do.

Keep a small palette in your kit so you can mix shades and products, either a professional palette or one from a good art department. Always go for a transparent or plain white palette.

A spatula is useful for adding cream, powder or gel products to the palette.

Tweezers have multiple uses, including hair removal, applying individual or strip lashes or for picking up adornments such as sequins or crystals.

Lash curlers can transform a look and enhance the shape of the eye no end. There are a variety of options.

Disposable applicators should be kept at hand for applying to other people, mainly mascara. Never double-dip your disposable mascara wand. Always use a fresh wand for each eye to prevent cross-contamination. Disposables can be purchased online in bulk if needed.

*Tip – We always use a Sharpie
pen to write the month and
year of purchase by the expiry
symbol of products.*

STORAGE

Good storage is vital to keep and transport your essentials hygienically and to ensure you can easily access what you need. First, let's look at make-up expiration dates. Old products can contain harmful levels of bacteria that can cause some pretty alarming infections.

Some liquids, such as moisturiser and foundation, are easy to spot when they are past their best. The packaging expands or has condensation marks and the content separates. Products which have a high level of water or natural plant derivatives are hot contenders for bacterial growth. Powders such as blusher and eyeshadow have a longer shelf life, but speed of bacterial growth will be increased by repeatedly using a contaminated brush or sponge.

Next to the ingredients listing you will see an opened jar symbol which will include a number followed by the letter 'M'. The 'M' stands for 'months'. For example, a product may have the symbol 9M. This means you should throw it out nine months after opening.

Don't keep your products in the bathroom. The heat and humidity presents the perfect breeding environment for bacteria. Likewise, don't be tempted to keep your products in the fridge. The extreme temperature affects the stability and performance of the ingredients.

OLD PRODUCTS CAN CONTAIN *HARMFUL LEVELS* OF **BACTERIA** THAT *CAN CAUSE* SOME PRETTY *ALARMING INFECTIONS.*

Keep skincare and make-up in a dark, cool location to maximise their shelf life. Mini storage drawers and units that have compartments to divide up your products, making it easy to view and select them. You can separate products into colour, brands or style (depending on how organised you are!).

Palettes are the best way of coordinating and selecting your colours, either pre-stocked with colours or empty and magnetic, which you fill with your own pans of eyeshadows and blushers. These often have a transparent lid for ease of viewing. We like to label these to differentiate similar colours.

Lipstick shades are often the most frustrating products to locate when jumbled in your bag. We have found the easiest way to store these is with the use of plastic pill cases. These have compartments into which you can decant lipsticks and label. We use a different case for every variety – reds, corals, pinks, etc. This makes life so much easier!

Professional cases can often be quite pricey. For years we have used a medium-sized suitcase with wheels and an extendable handle. We separate our products into transparent zip-up bags for ease of access.

Brush belts are great for working in the industry. Working on location you will often find yourself in a dimly lit room or under fluorescent lights which alter the colour of your products. You can purchase your own portable lighting online. The kits fold down to a manageable size. The light bulbs replicate natural day-light and will illuminate the face and make-up to make your job a lot easier.

BRUSHES

These have become popular with consumers in the last ten years. Maybe this has something to do with the rise of social media channels such as Pixiwoo, where people can see how to use them.

Good brushes are not cheap, but they are an absolute necessity for longevity and precise application. Of course, the warmth of your fingers can be a great help when blending creams and liquids but brushes are the key to an immaculately executed look.

The confusingly large range of brushes can be categorised into two main types by bristles: synthetic and natural-hair.

Synthetic bristles are usually made of tacklon or nylon fibres. The bristles feel slightly more coated and have more of a sheen. The bristles are less porous meaning that cream, liquid and gel product will remain on the tips, allowing a longer play time.

GOOD BRUSHES ARE *NOT CHEAP,* BUT THEY ARE AN *ABSOLUTE NECESSITY* FOR LONGEVITY AND *PRECISE APPLICATION.*

Natural-hair brushes are made from a variety of hair types, often mixed, usually sable, pony, squirrel, badger, mink or goat. They feel flexible, soft and pick up more product while ensuring easy blending. They can be used with creams but perform better with powder.

The shape of the brush you select has a huge impact on the finish of your make-up and there are a bafflingly large number of styles available.

Fluffier brushes will lay down less product and create a very natural finish – good for blending or sweeping over products in a sheer wash.

Firmer, compact brushes pick up more product and allow for a precise application. Good for eyeshadow before blending or for creating a heavier impact. Looser, less compact brushes create a natural finish with foundation. A flat or firm brush will create a full, more flawless finish.

Blended or duo-fibre brushes mix natural and synthetic hair. They often appear darker (usually black) at the base and have white tips. Use with liquid or powder. The natural hair provides a firm base and holds extra product, while the synthetic white tips softly buff the product off the skin. Use product sparingly to avoid streaking.

Sponges can be used to apply base and are either latex or polyurethane foam (good for latex allergies). They give a buildable, smooth coverage and are often curved to make it easy to get to all the contours of the face.

THE *SHAPE* OF THE *BRUSH* YOU SELECT HAS A *HUGE IMPACT* ON THE *FINISH* OF YOUR *MAKE-UP.*

BRUSH CLEANSING

Dirty brushes harbour bacteria that cause skin infections or aggravate blemishes and acne. A brush full of old make-up will also shed hair, perform poorly and not last long.

Use a mild shampoo to clean make-up brushes and remove product residue. However, this has no anti-bacterial properties, so rinse the brush and then use a professional brush cleanser. Usually inexpensive, these are available in large quantities for multiple usage. They contain alcohol which kills bacteria and various proteins which help to condition and protect the hairs.

Clean your brushes at least three times a week if they are just being used on yourself and you have no skin conditions or blemishes. Otherwise, clean after every use.

First pour a small amount of cleanser into a glass and dip the brush in from the tips to halfway down the hairs.

Gently circle the brush onto a dry cloth or thick tissue to remove make-up. Be sure not to get the base of the brush hairs wet as this can loosen the glue which secures the hairs.

Ensure you reshape the brush hairs and leave them out to air-dry naturally either on their side or hanging upside down. Never stand them up straight to dry as water may seep into the glue at the base.

The alcohol in brush cleanser means hairs dry off quicker and you can use them again within a few minutes.

So, out of the hundreds of brush variations, which ones are essential?

DIRTY BRUSHES
HARBOUR *BACTERIA* THAT
CAUSE SKIN INFECTIONS
OR *AGGRAVATE*
BLEMISHES AND *ACNE.*

A GOOD *FOUNDATION BRUSH* CHANGES HOW *YOUR BASE LOOKS AND PERFORMS.*

This is often the hardest area to get right but get the skin correct and everything else will fall into place. A good foundation brush changes how your base looks and performs.

Flexible, looser-styled brushes are best for a sheer base of foundation that mimics your natural skin. Stippling brushes and duo-fibre brushes pick up less product and have a larger surface area to distribute product widely. Use a sweeping circular movement to buff the product into the skin, letting the tips of the brush do all the work. You can build product with this style of brush after the initial wash of colour has been buffed in.

Firmer, more compact brushes are best for medium-to-full cover. These have a more solid look and feel and are less flexible. They pick up more product and apply foundation in a condensed, smaller area, giving you a fuller cover. You can build and blend with this style of brush but keep a stippling brush at hand for the contours of the face.

Foundation brushes are synthetic or have synthetic tips. You can also use a real-hair brush but it will absorb more product.

Sponge coverage can also be altered. A damp sponge dilutes foundation slightly and helps to achieve a sheer finish. A dry sponge will give a fuller cover.

Concealer brushes are crucial to a flawless finish and come in different styles. Fluffy brushes are used on the delicate skin around the eyes or on slight colour discolouration. They buff the product in without dragging the skin and blend into your foundation seamlessly.

Firmer, flatter brushes are best for blemishes or areas which require a fuller cover. Use the flat of a synthetic brush to pat in the concealer and then the tip of the brush to blend the edges.

You can use both synthetic and natural-hair brushes on the eye area. You may prefer a synthetic brush with a cream and a natural-hair brush with powder, but in general, use a flatter, firm brush to lay down the initial product as it will push the product exactly where required. It is also great for building product and deepening tone.

Fluffy blending brushes are essential to blend a gradient of colour to perfection. Short-haired brushes will provide a dramatic blend and are good with products that require quick blending due to their fast drying time. A long, flexible-haired brush provides a softer blend. Product falls out a lot so be sure to give them a tap to remove excess powder before blending.

Some eye brushes are larger for quick application and to cover a broader area. Smaller eye brushes will be better for a smaller eye area or for more intricate colour placement.

Fine liner brushes or angled brushes are good for lining the eyes. The shorter the brush hair, the more control you will have over product placement. A more confident hand may prefer a longer, fine liner to create a sweeping feline flick.

Angled brushes are firmer and give better control over placement. The pointed end also helps you to create a sharper edge with your liner flick.

You can also use the same style of liner brush and angled brush on the brows. A double-sided brush comb is useful, with a firm bristle side to brush through brows and a fine tooth comb on the opposite side to separate lashes.

LIP BRUSHES

Some people prefer to apply their lipstick or gloss directly from the bullet. When applying to others it's more hygienic to use a lip brush. They are often retractable or have a case to cover the tip for transportation. Often these are synthetic brushes to avoid product absorption.

These are your larger powder, bronzer, contour and blush brushes and can be synthetic or natural-hair. The bigger the brush, the sheerer the finish. To achieve a good contour, use a firmer brush, ideally with an angle or squared-off edges, as they sit comfortably in the contours.

Kabuki brushes are short-stemmed with densely packed hairs and are commonly kept in the handbag for powder touch-ups.

THE *BIGGER THE BRUSH,* THE *SHEERER THE FINISH.* TO ACHIEVE *A GOOD CONTOUR,* USE A *FIRMER BRUSH,* IDEALLY *WITH AN ANGLE* OR *SQUARED-OFF EDGES,* AS THEY SIT COMFORTABLY *IN THE CONTOURS.*

Colour theory plays a huge part in the application of make-up and is often something that is overlooked when choosing tones and shades. There are no rules in make-up but it's a good idea to know a little background, especially when it comes to colour correction.

You may hear a lot of jargon used relating to colour theory and so we have broken down some of the popular terminology for you.

We have also created a colour wheel in the accompanying app. The colour wheel simplifies the information that follows so don't worry if at first this seems a little confusing!

Colour theory in make-up application usually divides into monochromatic and analogous looks:

Monochromatic is one colour applied and blended. The eyes, cheeks and lips are in varying tints, tones and shades. An example would be a brown smoky eye which blends into a lighter brown with a bronze blusher and a nude brown lipstick.

Analogous is a blend of two colours that sit next to each other on the colour wheel. The colours blend well with each other and are a good starting point to practise blending one colour into another. An example of this would be a blue eyeshadow that blends through to a green onto a yellow-green with a yellow highlighter.

We will go into much more detail on colour choice for the various areas of the face and body in the subsequent chapters but familiarise yourself with the colour wheel in the meantime.

HUE

The pure colour, e.g. green, blue and yellow.

VALUE

The lightness or darkness of a colour.

INTENSITY

The purity of the pigment. The brighter the pigment, the higher the intensity.

TINT

The pure colour plus white.

TONE

The pure colour plus grey.

SHADE

The pure colour plus black.

MONOCHROMATIC

A blend of one colour using any tint, tone or shade.

ANALOGOUS

Colours next to one another on the colour wheel
(a minimum of two but no more than five).

COMPLEMENTARY

Any two colours directly opposite each other on the colour wheel.
Opposite colours enhance one another.

PRIMARY COLOURS

Red, yellow and blue. Cannot be created by mixing.

SECONDARY COLOURS

Orange, green and violet. Can be created by mixing two primary colours.

TERTIARY COLOURS

Created by mixing one primary colour and one secondary colour.

WARM COLOURS

Have a red, orange or yellow undertone. These colours are also called
'advancing colours'. Advancing colours appear to project towards you.

COOL COLOURS

Have a green, blue or violet undertone. These colours are also known
as 'receding colours' and give a hollowed effect.

THE *SHORTER*
THE *BRUSH HAIR, THE*
MORE CONTROL…

...YOU *WILL*
HAVE OVER *PRODUCT*
PLACEMENT.

PIXI TIPS

[TOOLS]

1

Decant your lipsticks into cases for use on shoots. Twist your lipstick all the way up and, using a knife (be careful), slice the lipstick bullet off at the base and put it to one side. Use a brush handle to scoop the remaining lipstick from its plastic base. Put the scrapings into your palette pot and replace the original lipstick. You have the colour in your kit and you still have your lipstick to use on yourself!

2

Don't press your brush too hard. The hairs will splay out and be damaged.

3

Use less product if you get stripes in your foundation. Once blended, you can apply more product if needed.

SKIN

"Beautiful make-up starts with beautiful skin."

—————————— *Shu Uemura*

WE BELIEVE THE SKIN IS THE MOST
IMPORTANT AREA TO GET RIGHT. YOU
CAN HAVE THE MOST PERFECTLY BLENDED
EYESHADOW OR ACCURATELY PLACED
EYELINER BUT IF YOUR FOUNDATION DOES
NOT SIT WELL OR IS THE WRONG COLOUR
IT THROWS THE WHOLE LOOK OFF.

We often get asked what foundation is best for a dry, flaky skin or what foundation will give a flawless finish. Our answer to this is you need to get right back to basics and take a closer look at your skincare routine. If it doesn't suit the needs of your skin type then the best foundation in the world will not look perfect.

SKINCARE

Skincare is very subjective. We all read articles or listen to celebrity choices but everybody is different. You need to identify your own needs and adapt your routine to suit.

If you have zero idea of your skin type, then book a consultation with a skincare advisor. You should expect the therapist to enquire about your medical history, your diet, your general health, how your skin reacts in different situations, how it feels after washing, how it feels by the end of the day and how it feels in certain seasons, as well as about allergies, your current routine and your work environment.

They will establish why your skin could be dry or oily and what you are doing in response so that they can identify how they can help you. They will usually look at your skin under a magnifying lamp.

It's important to be honest. If you drink five cans of sugary drink a day, survive on four hours sleep a night and often sleep in your make-up then confess all! They can give you the best possible advice.

If a consultation is not an option then do a little research online. Most premium brands have interactive questionnaires. There are also some amazing skincare blogs, as well as various YouTube channels (including our very own Pixiwoo), with unbiased reviews.

Yes, some skincare products can be expensive and they're not always the best. But if you spend money on an expensive pair of shoes once a month, then look at substituting that for a premium skincare product. If you work to a tight budget there are also great options available.

SKINCARE IS VERY *SUBJECTIVE*. WE ALL READ ARTICLES OR LISTEN TO CELEBRITY CHOICES BUT *EVERYBODY IS DIFFERENT*. YOU NEED TO IDENTIFY YOUR OWN NEEDS AND *ADAPT YOUR ROUTINE TO SUIT*.

After researching online, you can even make some products in your own kitchen!

Here is what to look out for when selecting your skincare.

[CLEANSERS]

FACE WIPES

We are always getting into trouble from our skincare-savvy friends about our face wipe abuse but it's something we are working on!

Don't get us wrong, face wipes do have a place but only really in an emergency. They don't give you a deep-down cleanse and are a major offender in blocking public sewage systems and filling landfill sites. Always dispose of them in the bin rather than down the toilet!

MICELLAR WATER

An alternative to the face wipe, micellar water was created in Paris for people to cleanse without having to use the harsh city water.

Relatively inexpensive, it can be purchased in smaller sizes for travelling or going to festivals. Massage it all over the face and around the eyes and remove with a cotton pad.

FACIAL WASH

We probably all began to use this in our teenage years as it's targeted at the younger market with promises of acne- or oil-reduction.

A fair number contain surfactants to ensure the cleanser foams up, giving that slightly stripped, tight feeling. Think how it feels to wash with soap – facial washes basically give the skin the same texture and can be quite drying.

They are not best for problematic or sensitive skin as they tend to strip the skin of its natural, protective oils. If your skin is naturally dry then don't even go there.

CLEANSING BALMS

Our personal choice (when we are not being lazy with a face wipe). Balms usually feel oily but don't make the skin oilier. They are often gentle enough to use over the eyes and on mascara too.

These need to be carefully removed – use warm water or a warm face cloth if they are particularly thick – otherwise they continue to work throughout the day. The oil in them will cause your make-up to break down and separate on the skin.

Using a balm cleanser has seriously amped up how our skin looks and is definitely worth the extra minute of effort it takes to use. We prefer Emma Hardie, Balance Me, Elemis and Eve Lom.

TONING

Toners are the next step after cleansing and often forgotten. They help to clarify the skin, remove dead skin cells, balance the skin and prepare for new product. We once thought you toned only to ensure your cleanser was removed, but it's actually important in resurfacing and conditioning the skin.

Toner is the perfect potion for a dry or dehydrated skin as it helps attract moisture. For dry or dehydrated skin, a spritz-on toner is also a great option. These feel refreshing, moisturise and also help your foundation to blend into any dry patches. If your skin is in the combination or oily spectrum then a toner will help to balance.

Exfoliating toners are great at combatting blemishes or acne. They help to renew the skin and remove the dead skin cells that cause blockages. Stacey, who works with us at Pixiwoo, swears by exfoliating toners and has seen a huge reduction in skin breakouts after using them.

Good toner brands include Liz Earle and Clarins for a dry skin, and Biologique Recherche and Pixi Glow Tonic for a combination or oily skin.

TONER IS *THE*
PERFECT POTION
FOR *DRY* OR
DEHYDRATED SKIN
AS IT HELPS *ATTRACT*
MOISTURE.

MASKS ARE A *TREAT* TO BRIGHTEN SKIN OR TO HELP SOOTHE STRESSED, *INFLAMED SKIN*.

If we are totally honest with you... this is the part of skincare that we suck at. We have a million reasons (read: excuses) why we don't indulge in exfoliators, masks and serums as often as we should. We have two children each and it's hard to make the time and we are lucky with our skin (mainly genetics) and find less is more.

Yet these extras can generally be a really positive inclusion. It's just all about finding what works for you. Exfoliating gives an instant oomph. It removes dull, dead skin and increases circulation to the upper layers, helping to bring fresh nutrients to the surface. Just don't overdo it or you will be left with broken capillaries and sensitive skin.

Always choose an exfoliator that contains manmade, synthetic beads, usually made from polyethylene. Exfoliators containing natural beads are usually made from fruit kernels and can scratch the skin, although some people prefer that rough texture.

Serums are fluid treatments which are much thinner than normal moisturisers and sink into the deeper layer of the skin to target your specific skincare needs. They are often anti-ageing but also work to help with your skin type, and issues such as redness, inflammation, luminosity, tissue damage and pigmentation.

Masks are a treat to brighten skin or to help soothe stressed, inflamed skin. Creamy masks are best for a dryer skin because they nourish and plump. Clay- or charcoal-based masks work well on a combination/oily skin type because they have great drawing properties. They pull up grime and bacteria, ensuring your pores are left clean and congestion-free.

MOISTURISERS/ NIGHT TREATMENTS

Some moisturisers make your skin look greasy and affect your foundation. Some moisturisers cause your foundation to bobble up and roll off the face.

We have both been outed by many friends in the industry (mainly skincare queen Caroline Hirons) about our love of moisturisers containing mineral oil. We know it's a cheap option but, having insanely dry skin, it helps our make-up to sit better when filming tutorials.

Moisturisers are personal. They help to rehydrate and give your skin the protection it needs to face the day. You can also get moisturisers with sun protection factor (SPF), which save you an extra step in the morning although it's not enough protection for lying out in the sun.

Skin pigmentation increases and becomes darker with sun exposure so by using a moisturiser with an SPF you are giving your skin extra protection and preventing an increase in pigmentation or skin sensitivity.

At night, amp up your moisturiser. We love to use an oil. These are suitable for all skin types and are actually most beneficial for an oily or problematic skin type. Fight oil with oil!

When creating tutorials for our channel we use brands such as Embryolisse and Oilatum because they give a good amount of slip to our dry skin in preparation for foundation. Generally, we recommend Clarins, Elemis, Sunday Riley, Estée Lauder, or budget options such as The Body Shop, La Roche-Posay and Boots No7.

[SKIN TYPES]

It can be difficult to identify your skin type without in-depth questions in order to make informed choices. We have certain questions we always ask our clients and you should consider them in choosing products. Use this tick box exercise – add up the ticks to determine your skin type:

DRY SKIN

- ☐ Redness or sensitivity
- ☐ Dry or flaky
- ☐ Flat and lacking radiance
- ☐ Tight after washing
- ☐ Lacking plumpness and elasticity
- ☐ Make-up clings to facial areas
- ☐ Visible capillaries

OILY SKIN

- ☐ Open pores
- ☐ Breakouts
- ☐ Shiny an hour after cleansing
- ☐ Make-up moves easily or pools in areas to give a curdled appearance
- ☐ Sensitivity
- ☐ Blackheads, especially around the nose and chin
- ☐ Dullness

SENSITIVE SKIN

- ☐ Easily aggravated by products
- ☐ Red or patchy
- ☐ Dry patches
- ☐ Reacts to weather or certain foods and drink
- ☐ Dullness
- ☐ Blackheads
- ☐ Thinness or visible capillaries

COMBINATION SKIN

- ☐ Oily T-zone
- ☐ Normal cheeks or slightly dry cheeks
- ☐ Open pores on nose and chin
- ☐ Occasional breakouts in the centre of the face
- ☐ Tight after washing
- ☐ Make-up slides off the centre of your face during the day
- ☐ Shine only around forehead and nose

STUDY *YOUR DIET* AND *RECOGNISE* WHEN IT *IS HAVING* A *NEGATIVE* EFFECT ON *YOUR SKIN.*

In addition to asking questions we also feel the skin and do a quick visual check to see if there are open pores or any pigmentation, as well as push the skin up to test for fine dehydration lines.

Skincare is something we have become better at identifying and applying but we believe a lot of it is genetic.

Our mum, Judy, has fabulous skin and so does our nan. But if you're not as lucky with your type, it just means you need to think more about what you are applying and you have to treat your skin kindly.

Look at your diet. Allergies and what you put into your body have a huge influence on your skin.

Eating a rainbow of fruit and veg is important. Leafy greens, such as spinach and kale, are great antioxidants and vitamin C improves collagen levels, so ensure you're eating plenty of fruit as well as vegetables such as sweet potato and broccoli.

Oily fish helps to give the skin a moisture boost and aids suppleness.

Drink up to two litres of still water a day.

Vitamin and fish oil supplements can help.

Study your diet and recognise when it is having a negative effect on your skin. Sugar is a hot contender for causing breakouts, as is caffeine, and for some people, dairy. Identify your aggressor and try to cut back but always consult your GP before making huge dietary changes.

Hormones have an absolutely massive impact on skin. At certain times of the month, the contraceptive pill and medication can affect hormones, but, again, be sure to consult your GP before making any changes.

SKIN TYPES HAVE CHARACTERISTICS THAT YOU CAN IDENTIFY.

DRY SKIN

- Often feels extremely tight after washing
- Appears matte with little or no shine
- Fine lines are more apparent
- Skin tone can look uneven
- Skin flushes easily
- Dehydrated (though we are pretty much all dehydrated due to the environment we live in)
- Flat and dull
- Sallow
- Oily and dry (oil on dry skin can be down to incorrect product choice leaving a film on the skin)

NORMAL SKIN

Generally well balanced with no dryness or oiliness, though we really don't think anyone has 'normal' skin; everyone has different elements.

COMBINATION SKIN

- Dry cheeks with an oily T-zone
- Open pores
- Can appear dull in places
- Blackheads and blemishes

Use balm cleansers to gently cleanse rather than strip the skin and acid toners that contain salicylic or glycolic acid. These help slough away dead skin to reveal a brighter complexion and help to prevent blemishes.

OILY SKIN

- Shine throughout the day
- Make-up will pool in areas or separate
- Flaky patches
- Open pores
- Blemishes

Use balm cleansers to nourish and hydrate but gently cleanse without stripping acid toners to remove build-up of dead skin cells that block the pores and lead to blemishes.

SENSITIVE SKIN

- Redness
- Tightness
- Uneven tone
- Easily aggravated

Use a gentle non-foaming cleanser, such as a milk or balm, to moisturise and calm. Use a lighter moisturiser that contains naturally healing ingredients such as aloe vera and camomile and natural oils such as neroli, rose or almond oil.

By identifying your skin type and appropriate skincare products, you will find selecting your base make-up products easier. Products will blend better, last longer on the skin and will enhance rather than mask your beautiful skin.

SKIN BREAKOUTS AND ACNE

Our clients and models often say, 'Oh, my skin is awful, I'm so spotty.' Nine out of ten times their skin has only one or two tiny, red bumps. These annoying spots normally arrive on a day when you need to look your best, but please know that everyone else is too consumed with how they look themselves to notice. We all get them.

Do wash your face with a suitable cleanser and follow a good skincare routine but remember that over-washing with harsh products can dry the skin to the extent that it compensates with more oil.

Don't pick at spots. They never dry up and heal. When you squeeze out the fluid, the bacteria spreads elsewhere and you are left with a red, pulsating spot that forms a hard scab. This is harder to conceal than the original red, soft spot.

One-off blemishes can be related to hormones, diet or stress. We both get the occasional spot at the same time each month and almost always on the chin. This screams hormones. We use a topical spot treatment to help reduce the inflammation. Don't apply strong, alcohol-based products that sting.

Our favourite products are oil treatments containing benzoyl peroxide or blemish creams containing salicylic acid. They exfoliate the skin without drying or stripping. Exfoliating toners prevent future blemishes and also speed up healing time.

Acne is a medical condition. It's not just a breakout in teenagers – although, unfortunately, there are still some GPs who dismiss acne as insignificant. Many will prescribe appropriate topical or oral medications. Be persistent and don't feel you have to put up with it.

PRODUCT RECOMMENDATIONS
FOR PROBLEMATIC SKIN

Milk or balm cleansers (never foaming cleansers that strip the skin) and acid toners to eliminate dead skin cell build-up. Fight oil with oil and use a nourishing night oil on the skin.

Look for glycolic and salicylic acid and oils containing benzoyl peroxide. These reduce bacteria on the skin and moisturise, preventing skin from peeling around blemishes.

BODY CARE

Think about all visible skin, not just the face. The neck and the ears are often forgotten but always give the game away when they appear a different colour in photos.

On an editorial shoot or with a bride be sure to buff a little foundation and bronzer over the ears and onto the neck if necessary.

It's usually around May that we realise we will expose more of our limbs to the world and it does actually get pretty hot in the UK. MAC Face and Body foundation is a great water-based foundation for the arms and legs. We mix a little in with a body lotion and massage over the skin. It's transfer-proof, but it isn't water-resistant so be careful in humidity if you're wearing white!

OVER-WASHING WITH *HARSH PRODUCTS* CAN *DRY THE SKIN* TO THE EXTENT THAT *IT COMPENSATES* WITH *MORE OIL*.

SKIN DISORDERS AND INFECTION

Here are some of the skin conditions we have come across:

COLD SORES

Usually you'll feel the tingling on the lip before the cold sore appears. Immediately get an anti-viral cream from the chemist. Cold sore patches can protect the area while it heals.

Avoid wearing make-up on the area to allow it to heal or at least decant liquid concealer onto the back of your hand and gently dab over the area. Alternatively, try dark lipstick if the sore is on the lip area. Scrape lipstick onto a palette and apply with a disposable brush. Never apply directly from the lipstick bullet.

At the cosmetic counter, always get the consultant to sanitise the lipstick or lip liner before application to prevent infection. They will be more than happy to do this for you. Some brands have a beaker of Isopropyl alcohol for you to dunk lipstick.

CHICKEN SKIN AKA KERATOSIS PILARIS

We both suffered with this as teenagers and were regularly taunted (children can be so cruel!). This is red/purple, bumpy, pimply skin, usually in the backs of your arms or thighs. Keratin builds up in the hair follicles, blocking them and causing rough patches of spotty skin. It's commonly found in adolescent females. Quite often you inherit chicken skin from your parents but it usually occurs in people with fair, dry skin.

Ensure your diet contains lots of Omega 3 fatty acids. These can be found in walnuts, oily fish, salmon and veg such as Brussels sprouts.

Exfoliate your body two to three times a week or use exfoliating gloves in the shower. This loosens the keratin plugs and softens the skin. Slather on a body cream to keep the area soft and moisturised.

ECZEMA/DERMATITIS

We both suffered bouts of eczema as children and also had a recurrence during pregnancy – behind the knees, the crook of the arm and, weirdly, behind the ears. Some poor souls even get it on their eyelids. It causes itching and is worse during the summer months when these areas get sweaty.

One cause is lack of natural oil and stress can also play a huge part, as can dairy intolerance. Stacey at Pixiwoo had severe eczema as a child in reaction to cow's milk. In the early 1980s it was hard to get hold of alternative milk so her dad bought a goat from his mate down the pub (standard rural Norfolk) for its milk. She was cured!

These days a GP will prescribe topical emollients to keep the skin supple. Steroids are also often prescribed to reduce flare-ups but should be used as a short-term measure. Keep the skin clean, dry and well moisturised.

Avoid over-exposure to sun or wind. Wear cotton nightwear to reduce sweating.

Dermatitis is a similar condition. Tons of our hairdresser friends suffer from it due to their constant hand washing and exposure to chemicals. Dermatitis is caused by irritants or allergic reactions. Quite often we have seen it as a result of contact with belt buckles, jean buttons, rings and metal arms of eyeglasses.

Avoiding the offending allergen or applying a layer of clear nail varnish to the backs of buttons or belt buckles can help. Steroid cream can be prescribed but a good rich lotion will help.

PSORIASIS

Psoriasis can be hereditary but can also be caused by the body overproducing skin cells. The skin can become layered and resemble dry, hard scales in severe cases.

Specialist skin emulsions help but a little exposure to the sun can also be beneficial. Vitamin D from sunlight is known to reduce the inflammation and help reduce symptoms.

For any extra information or help regarding these conditions you can check out the following websites:
www.nhs.uk
www.britishskinfoundation.org.uk
www.eczema.org
www.psoriasis-association.org.uk

THE EYES ARE THE FIRST FEATURE WE NOTICE. THEIR SHAPE, COLOUR, THE EYESHADOW COLOUR AND EYELINER FLICK. EYES ARE EXPRESSIVE AND OFTEN THE FIRST AREA TO SHOW SIGNS OF AGEING AND SUN-DAMAGE.

We were in our twenties when we began posting on YouTube and now we are in our late thirties we know there are visible changes to our eyes. We try to embrace them, just as everyone who wears make-up needs to make changes to their eye make-up over time. Frustration can occur when we try to apply the same products and techniques we used years ago. We all need to make a natural adjustment.

In this section we will help you select products, whatever your age, and also show you which textures, colours and finishes will benefit and enhance your beautiful eyes.

Tip – UV damage to the eyes and surrounding skin begins at an early age, so if you have young children get them some sunglasses.

SKINCARE FOR THE EYES

The skin around the eyes is very thin and fragile, approximately 0.5mm thick. It is constantly moving as we smile or speak and is exposed to the elements daily.

Lifestyle and diet play their part and can make this area grey, dull, puffy or dehydrated. If your mother or father have dark circles then, genetically, there's a high chance you will too. Healthwise, red, irritated eyes can indicate conditions such as hayfever or food allergies.

Sunglasses are your saviour. You may feel like a bit of a diva wearing them on a dull day but they provide the best protection for the delicate eye area. Winter or summer, we always have a pair – in our handbags, in the car or balanced on our heads.

Look for complete UVA/UVB protection in choosing your sunglasses. 'Fashion sunglasses' may not give you the protection you need, so be sure to check the level of block. The bigger the sunglasses, the larger the area you protect. Choose a style that sits snugly and covers the area under the eyes too.

Eye creams get mixed reviews and are quite expensive. They come in tiny pots yet promise you renewed skin around the eyes. But quite often they have similar ingredients to your regular moisturiser alongside the cooling ingredients they use to help soothe the eye area.

If the skin around your eyes is simply dehydrated, with fine lines, then a small amount of your daily moisturiser or night treatment around the eyes is a cheaper and effective alternative.

We are rubbish at remembering to apply our skincare products and rarely get them. When we do use an eye cream we tend to go for one that illuminates. These have a light, balmy texture and are infused with super-fine, reflective particles to bounce the light off dark circles. We like to mix a little of the cream with our under-eye concealer and then apply as normal.

If it's puffiness of the skin around your eyes that concerns you then use a lightweight eye gel or an eye cream with a metal applicator ball. The metal feels cool on the skin and temporarily reduces puffiness. Using these roller balls before make-up application also helps your make-up products to sit better.

Tap on eye cream with your ring finger, which has the lightest pressure and won't drag the delicate skin. Gently pat the product around the bony socket of the eye, taking it around the brow bone and into the side of the nose. The patting motion stimulates the circulation, bringing fresh nutrients to the skin and helping to shift toxins around the eye area.

We have found cooling gel patches to be really beneficial. We love the ones made by Skyn Iceland but there are others available. These patches have a jelly-like texture and are pre-cut into a half-moon shape to fit comfortably under the eye. Infused with various cooling and calming ingredients, they will feel amazingly reviving on a stressed-out eye area.

We spend a lot of time in front of computer screens and are constantly removing and re-applying our make-up, so these are a godsend. Take ten minutes out with these on and you have an instant pick-me-up with visible results.

WE LIKE TO *MIX A LITTLE EYECREAM WITH* OUR *UNDER-EYE CONCEALER* AND THEN *APPLY* AS *NORMAL.*

YOU *CAN ALSO MAKE USE* OF YOUR *HOUSEHOLD* CULINARY *INGREDIENTS* TO CREATE *NATURAL REMEDIES.*

1

Coconut oil is great for conditioning hair and as an intensely moisturising night oil.

2

Mix oatmeal with almond oil as a body exfoliator.

3

Mash up an avocado with honey and plain yogurt to create a nourishing mask for all skin types. Slather on for ten minutes and wash off.

4

Use raw potato slices on the eyes to cool and tighten the skin. They stay cooler longer than cucumber or cooled tea bags.

DARK CIRCLES

We are often asked how to eliminate dark circles. Colour correction, foundation and concealer will help to cover the problem but you need to also look at underlying conditions:

1

Genetics (thank your parents). There isn't much you can do about this. Clever use of concealer is your best weapon.

2

Thin skin under the eye can reveal fine blood capillaries, creating a bluish tinge. Gentle under-eye massage can pep up the circulation and get the blood flowing. Use light tapping movements or pressure-point massage. Massage the under-eye area in a light, circular motion, working inwards to the nose.

3

Lack of sleep. Blood vessels under the eyes dilate when you're tired, causing a darker appearance. Reach for your cooling eye patches or eye gels. And try and get your eight hours of sleep if possible.

4

Dehydration. We always try and drink two litres of pure, still water a day. Not only will you see the results in your general appearance, but it also flushes out toxins around the eye that may be causing darkness. Water also helps with tiredness.

5

The ageing process. As we age the skin around the eyes becomes thinner and the eyes can appear more sunken. Eyelids become hooded and cast a shadow over the eye. Use eye creams as part of your skincare routine and follow our tips on applying make-up to a hooded eye.

6

Illness and medication. Unfortunately, illness often manifests itself in our skin. Certain medication can also have an effect on our circulation and healing. Try facial massage and use a light, reflective eye cream. Check with your doctor before trying anything new, as massage can be over-stimulating.

EYE MAKE-UP REMOVER

We know that removing your eye make-up is the biggest chore when you're tired, but it's something you must do. It not only cleanses delicate skin around the eye but also prevents product flaking into the eye while you sleep and potentially scratching the surface.

EYE MAKE-UP WIPES

Some people use a regular face wipe but these may sting the eyes. Purpose-made eye wipes are much smaller and contain ingredients that calm and soothe the area.

BI-PHASE REMOVERS

These should be used for heavy eye make-up. One layer is oil-based and a second layer is usually water-based and has other soothing ingredients.

After a good shake, the two layers mix to create an oily substance that lifts off all, even water-resistant and waterproof products. Massage this over the eyes and then remove with a cotton pad. Don't use between make-up applications as it can leave an oily film and you will struggle to get products to stick to the skin afterwards.

LOTION/CREAM REMOVERS

Cream or lotion removers are great for most types of make-up. They can feel quite rich on the skin so work well on dry, dehydrated or mature skin. Massage over and remove with a cotton pad.

COTTON BUD SWABS

These are like standard cotton buds (or Q-tips) but are infused with eye make-up remover. You usually have to snap a seal to release the remover into the cotton bud. These are great both for removing eyeliner and for correcting mistakes.

PRIMERS

Skin primers create a barrier between the natural oils and texture of your skin and foundation. We only wear them when we have no time to touch up our make-up or we are in a hot/humid environment.

Working on a shoot, editorial work or at a fashion week we rarely use a primer. We have to create multiple looks or adapt make-up and primer makes alterations and removal more difficult.

When doing one-off make-up application for events such as a wedding, prom or red carpet event, primers help with longevity. The finish is smoother for skin with open pores or fine lines.

Use sparingly with a duo-fibre brush or stippling brush to ensure a light application. Apply too much and you'll find your foundation bobbles up and rolls off your face.

Work primer well into the skin and leave for a minute before applying foundation. Rather than

eye primers and lip primers we prefer eye pencil liner, a cream eyeshadow or a lip liner.

FOUNDATIONS

It's an absolute minefield choosing a foundation and just when you think you've found the perfect one it gets discontinued. It's worth paying for a good one.

Spending £5 will get you a chalky foundation with zero longevity and odd colour options. Select texture and coverage before colour. Take into consideration your skin type and coverage needed.

FOUNDATION FOR DRY SKIN

This needs to be able to blend and provide hydration and moisture with an adaptable coverage. You need to be able to sheer the foundation over areas of patchy skin so that it doesn't

SKIN *PRIMERS* *CREATE*
A *BARRIER* *BETWEEN*
THE NATURAL *OILS* AND
TEXTURE OF *YOUR* *SKIN*
AND *FOUNDATION*.

★

cling. A luminous or radiant finish foundation will sit well and feel comfortable. Liquid foundations have more fluidity to blend in.

Cream foundations give a great radiance and feel comfortable on the skin but cling to patches and sit in dehydration lines. Silicone-based foundations give a beautiful finish but we find the silicone clings to a dry skin.

Facial spritz is a water-based spray you can either use directly on your face or your foundation brush. It helps to blend foundation into dry areas or over patchy skin. Powder foundations are a no-no. They absorb moisture and will cake and crack.

Get wise to the ingredients in your foundation. The higher up the ingredients are listed, the larger their quantity. Aqua and glycerine are good ingredients in the top five.

FOUNDATION FOR COMBINATION SKIN

Combination skin is probably the hardest foundation to suit due to the mix of textures. Cheeks are often dry so need a little moisturisation and the T-zone is oily so a matte texture is required.

You don't need a matte finish for a little skin shine. You may want radiance in areas but just matte in the centre panel of the face. To achieve this, you need multiple products.

If you want a matte finish all over then a liquid foundation will be a safe option. Dust a powder over the centre of the face to absorb any oil if needed.

Powder foundation will also work on combination skin requiring a matte finish but you need the correct colour. As the powder mixes with the oils in the skin they often darken. This is called oxidisation. Combat this with primer or by opting for a slightly lighter colour than your skin tone.

You can then go in with a bronzer to warm the skin tone up. For a radiant finish use a matte primer on the T-zone and a satin finish foundation. Use a translucent powder on the T-zone and a cream or liquid highlighter on the high points of the face to add radiance.

FOUNDATION FOR OILY SKIN

The biggest problems are longevity and colour. Product pools or slips quicker and the foundation oxidises and changes colour.

Have patience and put in the prep work. Let's assume you have your perfect skincare routine in place...

Give your moisturiser a few moments to sink in. Apply an oil-free primer (silicone varieties work well on an oily skin).

Using a stippling brush (sheer cover), or a firm, chunky foundation brush (full cover), apply a small amount of liquid foundation and buff well. Apply your concealer if required.

Leave your base for a good five minutes while you complete the rest of your make-up to allow the foundation to move and settle.

Check any areas that may need buffing in again and then powder.

Press your powder into the skin with a velour pad and then apply any bronzer, etc.

Always expect to have to touch up during the day – but at least the main base will remain.

Powder foundations will give you an instant matte finish. You can still layer with a primer first and add concealer before application.

Never keep your powder foundation sponge/pad in the compact. The oil (and bacteria) from your pad will transfer into the product, causing the powder to harden and develop a film or seal.

Choosing your correct foundation shade will make or break your look. It's one of the hardest things to get right. The brands don't make it any easier to figure out.

Each company uses a different scale to grade their foundation colours. Most brands will tend to have either yellow- or pink-based foundations.

Yellow-based foundations look golden and warm in the bottle. They tend to suit more sallow skins, people who tan easily or olive skin tones.

Pink-based foundations look cooler and ashier-toned in the bottle. They suit much fairer skin tones or people who get any redness.

Quite often both undertones will suit your skin and it's just a case of deciding which you prefer.

Darker skins may need a pink base around the mouth and hairline while the rest of the face needs a yellow base.

If using two foundations is not an option then use a foundation which will suit the predominant colour and go in with a concealer in the opposite colour tone on the areas which are a different colour.

SKIN TONE CHECKLIST

- Obvious yellow or pink undertone to cleansed face
- Red undertone to chest to blend with the skin tone
- Areas requiring yellow or pink bases
- If wrist veins appear green then skin tone is warmer and requires more of a yellow base. If veins appear blue then the skin will be pink-based.
- Still confused? Swipe your closest shade in both yellow and pink onto the face and blend. The one that blends away invisibly will work best.

[SKIN]

CHOOSING YOUR *CORRECT FOUNDATION* SHADE WILL *MAKE OR BREAK* YOUR LOOK. IT'S *ONE OF* THE *HARDEST THINGS* TO *GET RIGHT.*

Tip – Take a little of your normal foundation over the top if needed, but it may affect the water resistance of the camouflage cream.

FOUNDATION FOR MATURE SKIN

As the skin matures, fine and deeper set lines begin to appear and you need to be more careful in the texture of your products.

Moisturising liquid foundations, which have a soft radiant finish, are a safe bet. Look for hydrating sheer foundations or bases which contain hyaluronic acid to plump the skin. Avoid anything too heavy or cream-based that sits in lines and exaggerates them.

If you like powders, pick a very fine, pressed product, patting it into the skin well and only applying it to areas of shine.

If your skin flushes easily then try a hydrating primer which has a slight green tint. Use this sparingly under your foundation and buff in well.

A skin-calming facial spritz cools and reduces high colour. Spritz this onto your make-up brush when applying your foundation to aid blending, but also spray over the face throughout the day as needed.

CONCEALER

Cream concealers are thicker and provide a better cover. They are good for blemishes, scarring and pigmentation. Use sparingly and build up using a flat, synthetic concealer brush or a very fine, firm detail brush for smaller areas.

Liquid concealers are better around the eyes and for areas that require less cover. They are thinner so won't settle and crease as much in fine lines. Use with a fluffy blending brush to push into the skin.

Don't confuse highlighting concealer pens with regular concealers (think YSL Touche Éclat). These give radiance rather than conceal and will leave you with those classic panda eyes in photographs. Use them to add natural highlights.

COSMETIC CAMOUFLAGE

Camouflage make-up should be used to cover acne, birthmarks and other skin pigmentation, vitiligo, rosacea, chloasma and tattoos.

It provides complete cover and even skin colour while protecting the skin underneath and is usually water-resistant or waterproof. A normal concealer will not perform as well over areas that require strong coverage.

We recommended waiting six months post-surgery before applying on scars to ensure the area has healed.

Camouflage creams are dermatologically tested and suitable for all skin types. Any age can use them and they usually come in a vast colour selection. These specialist products are often only available to purchase online or in selected salons. Most brands offer a sample kit containing a selection of shades. They also include small vials of the finishing powders and colour correcting powders to set the cream. Make-up artists should keep a kit in each colour in case a job requires it.

Camouflage creams are very thick and only require a small amount of product. Ensure skin is moisturised before applying the camouflage cream directly onto the skin using a cosmetic sponge with a rolling action. You don't need much pressure if the area is sensitive.

Give the cream a good few minutes to sink in and adhere to the skin. Buff the edges with a soft blending brush. We then like to apply regular foundation to the rest of the face and buff this into the edges of the colour correction patch. Dust over the specialist powder to set the cream with a large, soft brush and pat the powder over the area rather than buffing. For tattoos, use the colour wheel to select the opposite colour for toning down the majority colour.

To knock back the black or ashy grey-toned outlines, apply a soft peach or orange first in

*Tip – If we are covering
a tattoo we use a colour-
correcting product underneath
the camouflage cream.*

a small quantity. If the tattoo has a lot of green or blue then apply an orange or red first. Use a regular colour corrector if possible but a lip liner or lipstick in red or orange will work well. Buff a small amount over the tattoo and sponge on your camouflage cream.

Good brands to check out for specialist cosmetic camouflage are: Keromask, Dermablend and Veil Cover cream.

CONCEALING BLEMISHES

Concealing blemishes is totally different to slapping on a bit of under-eye concealer and blending with your finger. You need to prep the skin, work hygienically and be precise with your colour and technique.

Blemishes are hard lumps under the skin. Unless picked or annoyed they are smooth, but red, hot and slightly raised. Nothing will make them appear flat so you just have to work on toning down the redness.

Remember hideous woodchip wallpaper? If you paint over the woodchip you will still see the knobbly, bumpy texture underneath. To get a smooth wall you need to remove the bumpy texture first. It's the same with bumps on the skin.

CONCEALING BLEMISHES
IS TOTALLY *DIFFERENT*
TO *SLAPPING ON* A BIT
OF *UNDER-EYE CONCEALER*
AND *BLENDING* WITH
YOUR FINGER.

YOU NEED TO GET YOUR SKINCARE RIGHT BEFORE YOU INVEST IN FOUNDATION:

1

Apply foundation as normal.

2

Use a cream concealer on a firm, flat brush and push a minimal amount of the concealer onto the spot using the flat of the brush.

3

Use a clean, fluffy brush to blend the edges into the skin. Build the concealer up if necessary.

4

Leave for a few moments and then apply a small amount of loose powder on a small brush. Dab the powder on.

5

Concealing a blemish covered with dry skin or a scab needs a little more work.

6

Apply your moisturiser and blemish treatment and allow them to sink in.

7

Use a small, soft brush, such as an eyeshadow blending brush, to apply your foundation over the area.

8

You can give the area a spritz with a facial water spray and use this moisture to blend the foundation.

9

Grab a cream concealer and, using a fine, firm eye lining brush, apply the concealer in tiny, delicate strokes to any areas of redness.

10

Touch up through the day if necessary. Avoid powdering a dry blemish with a scab as the moisture in the skin will be absorbed and powder adheres to dry patches.

It's super-important to use a clean brush on the blemish. Clean and sanitise your brush after use.

POWDER

Powder helps to mattify the skin and set the foundation and concealer under-neath but it's not a necessity.

Loose powder has a natural finish. A good powder releases a plume of fine powder when you open the lid. Control application with a small dusting brush to specific areas.

Pressed powders are great to keep in your bag for touch-ups. They tend to give a sheer to medium cover. Apply with a pad and remember to turn your pad over if storing in the palette case to avoid oil transferring into the powder and causing a seal.

Blot powders are colourless or have a small percentage of colour pigment and don't oxidise. These are great for very oily skin, removing shine but don't colour or cover.

COLOUR CORRECTORS

These are great for rosacea or flushing (naturally, menopausal or after alcohol/ spicy food). They pep up a dull skin, tone down ashy, dark circles or neutralise a sallow skin.

Good colour correcting will create a veil over natural tones, helping them to blend in naturally. Kind of like using a photographic filter.

USE MINIMAL AMOUNTS AND BLEND WELL

Apply liquid primer style colour corrector after moisturiser and before your foundation. Buff with a stippling brush over the areas required. Alternatively, blend a pea-sized amount with your moisturiser.

Apply cream colour corrector under your foundation or mix a little in with your regular concealer and use it on top.

Apply powder colour corrector by dusting lightly. A pink, loose powder is particularly good at toning down yellow foundation.

Use our colour wheel to choose the tone of colour corrector. Look at the colour you are trying to hide on the wheel and then look to the opposite side for the balancing colour. For example, dark grey or purple circles under your eyes are balanced by a warm, peach- or yellow-based corrector.

PRESSED *POWDERS*
ARE *GREAT* TO
KEEP IN *YOUR BAG*
FOR *TOUCH-UPS*.

COLOUR CORRECTION GUIDE

USE GREEN FOR:

- Toning down red/pink blemishes
- Rosacea
- Scarring
- Skin flushing
- Allergic skin

USE ORANGE/PEACH FOR:

- Grey or purple dark circles
- Bruising
- Giving radiance to a darker skin tone
- Lifting an ashy/dull skin tone

USE YELLOW FOR:

- Brightening a pale ashy skin tone
- Use as an eyeshadow base on a veiny eyelid

USE PINK FOR:

- Brightening a lighter skin tone
- Faded bruises with a green/yellow undertone
- Ashy patches on a medium skin tone

USE PURPLE OR LAVENDER FOR:

- Sallow/yellow skin tone
- Times when you have been ill and need a boost
- Evening out a patchy tan

Tip – For oily skin, if you prefer not to use powder at all then paper blotting sheets are great. They often come in a handy-sized packet with small sheets of highly absorbent paper to absorb oil on the face. They don't disturb your base make-up and won't leave residue.

Tip – For feet and backs of hands, mix a small amount of tan with your body lotion to thin the product out.

TANNING

We are all aware of the dangers of the sun and tanning beds. Fake tans are a great alternative but we have seen some pretty obvious disasters. Orange patches on the elbows and heels, orange fuzz on the chin, streaky legs and tanned palms are the main offenders.

Most fake tans work in the same way: you apply, leave them on for a few hours and then shower off. Never apply and then go out for the evening! It's gross, it stinks, it develops throughout the night and if it rains then you're screwed. It can also stain clothes.

Salon tanning is good if you're short of time or just don't want to risk getting it wrong. It's possibly one of the most ridiculous situations you will find yourself in; naked except for a pair of see-through paper knickers and a shower cap, legs spread and arms up, all in front of a total stranger. The worst bit is when they ask you to turn around and hoist your bum cheeks up to get to the patch which is obviously covered by your sagging cheeks! It takes minutes though, and they are always super-professional and discreet.

If driving, park close to the salon and wear flip-flops to avoid marking your feet. Take a bin bag to sit on for your drive home to avoid staining your car seat. When you leave, dressed in some hideous, loose tracksuit, you can guarantee you'll bump into someone you know. If that all sounds too traumatic then purchase your own fake tan and have a go.

GRADUAL TANNERS

These are great to start with. Just like an ordinary body lotion, you apply in the morning or evening and it will slowly give you a tint to your skin throughout the week. Control the level of tan by applying every day or every other day. Gradual liquid tanners mix with your face moisturiser to give you sun-kissed skin.

LIQUIDS

These are runny, usually tinted on application and are easily splashed onto the floor or curtains. They sneakily run down the back of your legs without you realising.

Tip – Mix your normal body lotion, diluting the strength, but giving more substance and blending more easily.

*Tip – Remember,
fake tan always looks
better two days
after application!*

MOUSSE

Easy to handle and massage. You need to use a lot as it doesn't spread far. We find it dries quickly so apply and blend quickly.

SPRAYS

Good at getting to the hard-to-reach areas but also hard to control. Best applied standing in the shower with the door closed.

At least 24 hours before applying tan, exfoliate your body and face. Concentrate on heels, elbows and any dry skin. Slather on body lotion and really work it into the elbows and knees.

Think about where you would tan naturally: don't apply too much to the underside of the forearms or armpits. You can use a gadget which looks like a bathing loofah on a long handle to reach your back and bottom.

Select your tan and, using a tanning mitt, begin to apply to the body in sweeping, circular move-

ments. Apply just before you go to bed to develop while you sleep. The downside is that you never get a good night's sleep. Fake tan seems to make you sweat more.

Lay an old towel over the pillow and bed sheet and sleep in loose-fitting old clothes or under a dressing gown to avoid transfer of product. Shower off in the morning and apply lots of moisturiser.

SUN PROTECTION

For centuries, a tan was seen as something the lower classes had – those who had to be outside or ploughing the fields were tanned from their work. It's only since the 1920s that it became a desirable look.

Sun protection needs to be instilled from a young age. Most of the sun exposure we receive in our lifetime happens before we hit our twenties.

YOUR *SUNSCREEN SHOULD PROTECT YOU* FROM *BOTH* UVA AND *UVB RAYS.*

New regulations and changing medical advice can be confusing, so here are our tips:

Your sunscreen should protect you from both UVA and UVB rays. UVA (Ultra Violet A) rays penetrate through to the deeper layers of the skin. They damage the cells deep within. These rays tan and, unfortunately, are also linked to skin cancer and skin ageing.

UVB (Ultra Violet B) cause the agonising sunburn you see a lot of Brits sporting as soon as the sun makes an appearance.

Apply a minimum of SPF 15 (UVA/UVB). Don't be stingy. You need a lot more than you think and need to re-apply at least every two hours. Alternatively, look for brands that require just one application for up to ten hours.

For a combination or oily skin type, you should opt for a specialist facial sunscreen. If you are not sunbathing, a primer or foundation with added SPF will often be enough.

PIXI TIPS

[SKIN]

1

If you are unsure about foundation, go lighter as, generally, they warm up a little on the skin. It's easier to darken a foundation with bronzer than it is to lighten it.

2

Forgot to wash your hands after applying fake tan? Squeeze the juice of a lemon into a bowl and add in a little salt. Scrub this mixture all over your hands to help bleach out the staining naturally. This will sting if you have cuts on your hands.

3

A make-up stippling brush can stand in for a tanning mitt. Clean your brush thoroughly afterwards.

4

Mix a little of your cream or liquid highlighter with your body cream and apply to the shoulders and shins to create definition.

5

Oil from your skin can transfer onto your phone. Each time you press the phone onto your cheek you are applying a layer of bacteria back onto the skin. Give your phone a clean over each day to avoid this.

FINISHES

*"The most beautiful make-up of a woman is passion.
But cosmetics are easier to buy."*

———————————— *Yves Saint-Laurent*

WE *OFTEN FEEL* THAT OUR *MAKE-UP DOESN'T COME TOGETHER* UNTIL WE HAVE A *TOUCH OF BRONZER* OR *BLUSHER* TO MAKE US *LOOK ALIVE* AGAIN!

FINISHES PULL YOUR WHOLE LOOK TOGETHER. POWDER DUSTED ONTO THE SKIN, BLUSHERS AND CONTOURING PRODUCTS FIT INTO THIS CATEGORY. WE OFTEN FEEL THAT OUR MAKE-UP DOESN'T COME TOGETHER UNTIL WE HAVE A TOUCH OF BRONZER OR BLUSHER TO MAKE US LOOK ALIVE AGAIN!

FACE POWDER

Powder has been around for thousands of years. In ancient Egypt, women would use clay-based yellow ochre powder to give their faces a matte but golden appearance. Japanese geishas combined rice powder and water to create the thick, white paste for that blanked-out white face. And archae-ological digs continue to unearth ancient, ornate powder compacts used by wealthy women and men.

There is now so much choice in powder types that it's hard to know where to begin. But while considered a must-have, it's often over-used or even completely unnecessary. Powder can enhance your skin, but it can also make your make-up noticeably heavy and highlight skin texture.

WHEN TO USE POWDER

If you have dry skin, note that powder absorbs moisture, but can help with base make-up longevity. Use very fine and loose powder – it releases a deli-cate plume of smoke-like particles when you open the container.

Use a large powder brush, lightly dusting the product. Applying too much will dry the skin and gives you a duller finish. Powders with a radiant finish sit more comfortably on dry skin. Avoid applying over extremely dry skin and where there are fine or dehydration lines.

Powder is most beneficial on a combination or oily skin. It mattes the skin, absorbs excess oil and controls make-up movement.

Apply sparingly and be cautious with your colour choice, otherwise your skin ends up caked in powder that looks congealed and makes you feel you need to give your face a wash!

We receive lots of emails from people saying their powder looks almost curdled. Some powders contain too much talc or you may be over-applying.

Make sure you are using the right skincare for your skin type. Avoid foundation and concealer that is too moisturising and creamy. You can't eliminate oil entirely (and at least you won't wrinkle) but do apply thin layers of skincare, primer and foundation, with a sheer veil of powder to keep it all in place.

Use translucent (colourless) powder or select a powder a shade lighter than your natural skin tone. When powder mixes with the natural oils in your skin it oxidises and becomes slightly deeper throughout the day. It may give you an orange, patchy base... not a good look.

MAKE *SURE* YOU *ARE* *USING* THE *RIGHT* *SKINCARE* FOR *YOUR* SKIN TYPE.

LOOSE POWDER

We prefer loose powder over pressed simply because we both have dry skin and don't like too much cover or oil absorption. The pots are not very portable but look beautiful on your dressing table.

It's easy and hygienic to use loose powder with a large brush and dust over the skin but use a smaller setting brush for controlled use over a smaller, specific area or to avoid transfer to contact lenses. Use matte finish for oily skin or the fine pearl finish for dryer or dull skin. The powder reduces shine and prolongs your base make-up.

PRESSED POWDER

Pressed powder comes in a compact with a mirrored lid and powder puff. These are portable but not indestructible so do keep them in a protective make-up bag.

Pressed powders, applied with a powder puff or sponge, give a slightly fuller coverage than loose powders. A medium powder brush gives a sheer wash.

Don't store pads in your compact or at least make sure the surface faces the lid, otherwise oil from your skin sinks into the powder, forming a hard film.

Its bacteria will reduce the product's life and can lead to skin breakouts. Gently scrape off any film using the handle of your brush.

Translucent or coloured pressed powder varieties absorb oil, remove shine and are great for a combination skin type. Colourless blotting powder is good for particularly oily skin, providing a very sheer covering. It doesn't oxidise on the oil, change colour or curdle when layered throughout the day.

BRIGHTENING POWDER

Available in loose or pressed formula and usually infused with very delicate, light-reflecting particles. These can be ultra fine for a natural radiance or slightly chunky for a more extreme highlight. A lilac undertone will reduce yellowing and even out sallow-looking skin. Peach-based brightening powders lift a dull skin and balance ashy or grey undertones.

NATURAL INGREDIENTS HAVE *BECOME* STEADILY MORE *ATTRACTIVE* SINCE BRANDS BEGAN *LISTING* *THEIR INGREDIENTS* ON *PRODUCTS.*

The titanium and iron oxides often create a fine shimmer which isn't so good if you prefer a matte finish. They also flash back on camera, so avoid on your wedding day.

Natural ingredients have become steadily more attractive since brands began listing their ingredients on products. You can now get a mineral-based product for all areas of the face.

Iron oxides, titanium dioxide and zinc oxide are most frequently used, ground down to a very finely milled particle to form the powders' basis. Certain ingredients such as fragrance and preservatives are left out to prevent skin irritation.

We don't believe mineral products particularly help with acne, breakouts or sensitive skin but they shouldn't make the situation worse. Some brands claim they are so natural you could sleep in them but we would never recommend it.

Mineral powders feel lightweight and look sheer on the skin but the pigment, in our opinion, is never as strong or intense in colour as regular make-up.

BRONZING

This can be dangerous in the wrong hands! Think tactically – where would you naturally catch the sun? Chances are it would be the sides of the forehead, the bridge of the nose and across the top of the cheeks, the tops of the ears and maybe a little over the décolleté. This is where you should apply bronzer.

If you have fair skin, choose a bronzer in a natural beige. Don't go more than one or two shades darker than your natural skin tone and avoid anything too warm or orange-based. The darker your skin, the darker you can go.

Test in natural light before you purchase. Ask the retail artist to apply the bronzer and then step outside. Use a large powder brush for a sheer, natural finish. For cream bronzer, use a large, synthetic-tipped stippling brush in small, circular motions.

Pressed compact bronzers are easier to apply than loose powder. Cream bronzers provide the least mess. Bronzing pearls are a little old school and messy but they do give you a mixed blend of colours.

PRESSED COMPACT BRONZERS ARE *EASIER* TO *APPLY* THAN *LOOSE POWDER.*

CONTOURING

Applying powder or cream of a darker shade than your natural skin tone casts a shadow, making your face seem more structured and highlighting product is then applied to the high points of the face. A darker colour generally recedes an area while highlights enhance.

The overall effect subtly alters your features but you need to be realistic: it can't change your nose or give you Angelina Jolie's pout. It's best to use a gentle contour to emphasise your naturally beautiful features.

Contouring has been the biggest story in make-up over the last five years, but we think it's had its day.

Who decided that a structured cheekbone and an elongated nose was the perfect shape face anyway? Extreme contouring belongs on the stage or under bright lights on an editorial shoot.

CONTOUR PRODUCTS

Powders give a stronger contour, but we prefer creams as they can be blended to look more natural, are easier to use and, if you make a mistake, you can just buff the product off. We also prefer to use a cream highlighter as it gives a glossy radiance that never looks caked.

A *LIGHT TOUCH*
AND *THE CORRECT*
COLOUR CHOICE
ARE *ESSENTIAL*.

Tip —Strong, obvious contour never works well in daylight on the high street.

A light touch and the correct colour choice are essential. Don't go for a tan or deep brown contour colour but select a shade slightly deeper than your natural skin colour with a cool, grey undertone. Sounds bizarre? These colours are present in a shadow and are more realistic. Alternate between the application brush and a clean brush until you achieve a good blend. The correct brush selection makes a huge difference. These are our favourites:

1

Flat contour brush. Shaped like a letterbox in that they are long, slim and rectangular and used with powder products. Good for contouring large areas, such as the cheekbones, forehead or jawline. Place underneath the bone of the face and softly buff back and forth.

2

Thin, synthetic foundation brush. Pointed tip, great for cream products. Use the tip of the brush to apply your cream underneath the facial bones.

3

Angled, natural-hair brush. Bristles cut at an angled, soft gradient. Apply initial contour product, then use the angle to buff the powder into the skin and blend any hard edges.

4

Small, domed powder brush. For precision application of highlighter to high points of the face.

SKIN BAKING

This is a technique drag queens have used for decades but we would avoid it. While great under strong lighting it looks caked and shows up any fine lines or dryness around the eyes in daylight.

You create an intense highlight by applying a thick layer of light-coloured powder on the high points of the face and under the eyes. The warmth of the skin and the barrier created by the powder heats the foundation and helps it to set. Leave the powder for up to ten minutes to 'bake' or cook the foundation underneath. It also creates a lightened area of skin that is flawlessly covered.

STROBING

This new technique is a fresh approach to contouring and hard to get wrong. All you need are your illuminating products: cream highlighters, shimmering pearl liquids or light-reflecting powders.

After applying your normal base make-up, simply apply your highlighter to the high points of the face. Imagine a light bulb above your head, bathing all the higher areas of the face in light. This is where you need to apply your highlighter. You will push back the natural contours of your face without needing a dark contour and your skin will look radiant and healthy.

Don't overdo it, as you may look a bit sweaty. Before a night out, take a test photograph of your face with the flash on. If the highlighter reflects back too much, your face will look like a disco ball so, as always, use small amounts and build up!

BEFORE *A NIGHT OUT*, TAKE A *TEST PHOTOGRAPH* OF YOUR FACE WITH THE *FLASH ON.*

BLUSHER

Blusher is a product we usually apply last. It can transform a look, waking up the skin colour that has been blanked out by the base make-up.

Blusher should enhance your make-up and give your cheeks a flush of colour. We like to run a small amount through the socket of the eye to tie it all together nicely. First gently pinch your cheeks to make them flush before dusting on a little blusher. When the flush subsides you will have soft colour in the most natural position.

Just like eyeshadows, blushers come in a variety of different finishes:

MATTE BLUSHERS

These are the most natural, without shimmer or shine. They usually have a strong pigment, but can sometimes go a little patchy. Use a small amount and build up.

Matte blushers apply more easily over the top of powder as they cling to moisture. If you are using one over a creamy foundation, dust a little loose powder over the cheeks first to give you a base.

SATIN BLUSHERS

These have a silky texture and may give your skin a very natural reflection. Think of how a piece of satin fabric reflects the light. Suitable for all skin types and really easy to apply and blend.

SHIMMER BLUSHERS

This either has a fine, shimmering pigment to give a glow to the cheeks or contains chunky pieces of glitter. The larger the glitter, the more extreme the light reflection and the more metallic the look. Apply sparingly.

CREAM BLUSHERS

Apply to the apples of the cheeks for a sheer, rosy flush using a small, synthetic, duo-fibre brush in a circular motion. Alternatively, use your fingertips. Pat on the colour and the warmth of your fingers will blend the blusher. Apply a tiny amount and build up. It sits well on dry, normal or mature skin, but may slip quickly on oily skin. It'll wear off really fast if you frequently touch your face.

LIQUID BLUSHERS

Not so common, liquid blusher often comes with a small application brush in the lid. Dot on the liquid and give it a good blend with your finger or a synthetic brush. Work fast as liquid blusher dries super-fast and temporarily stains the skin.

BLUSHER *SHOULD ENHANCE* YOUR *MAKE-UP* AND *GIVE* YOUR *CHEEKS* A *FLUSH* OF *COLOUR.*

SETTING SPRAY

A setting spray is a fine mist that you can spritz over your completed make-up to help keep it in place. Use this rather than hairspray, which turns into a sticky film and can sting like crazy if you have sensitive or blemished skin. It's also not good for you to breathe in hairspray fumes or douse your face in the alcohol-laden spritz.

Most setting sprays are water-based and freshen the skin as you apply. They are also really useful to carry in case you find your foundation settles into fine lines or cakes during the day. Spritz over and re-buff your base for an instant refresh. We sometimes like to spray them onto our foundation brush to help blend our base product into the skin. They sheer out the foundation and prevent patchiness.

Setting sprays create a sheer veil and contain beneficial ingredients such as aloe and plant extracts. They form a fine barrier between your skin and the environment and also help prevent make-up transfer. If you have oily skin they will prolong your make-up's life as long as you are using the correct skincare and foundation. You also need to layer products in small amounts and remember all make-up is temporary as your skin sweats and moves.

PIXI TIPS

[FINISHES]

1 When it comes to powder, less is more.

2 Avoid applying powder over fine lines. It will enhance them and actually make them appear deeper.

3 Brush through your brows and lashes after applying powder to ensure no powder residue is caught in the hairs.

4 Use a powder to correct the look of your make-up if you feel that your base is a little too yellow. Dust a pink-based powder over the skin to knock back the sallow finish of your base. The pink also helps to brighten the skin colour.

5 Loose powder in a pot is easier to keep hygienic. Dispense the correct amount with the shaker-style lid. Make sure your powder brush is clean before dipping it into the pot. Remove the powder puff from the compact to keep your pressed powder hygienically.

6 Sanitising sprays are safe to spritz over all make-up, including powder products, but don't saturate. A gentle spritz from a distance is enough to kill the bacteria.

7 Contour by the window if you're preparing for the day or in a well-lit mirror for the evening.

First, we would like to say a massive thank you to all of our followers, who have supported us on this crazy and exciting journey. Without you it wouldn't be possible. X

Thank you: Gleam Futures, our fantastic management. You're the best of the best; it's rare to find managers that really and truly have the best interests of their clients at heart. You look after us so well. Dom, Francesca, Abigail, Viv and all the rest of the team, it's an absolute honour and pleasure to have your help and get to work with you daily. (Also, Sam apologises if anyone is ever offended by the overuse of swearing in her emails.)

Thanks to Dundas Communications: Max, Amy, Freya, Callum and Nancy, for helping to steer us in the best direction. Just like Gleam, you are a rare find.

Thanks to Blink for all your help with this book.

Thanks to our family: Mum, Ian, Steff, Danny, Brian, Lily, Ollie, Harry and Edie for supporting, entertaining and helping us along the way. Your positive attitude when times get hard always pulls us through and your help managing and juggling the children has been paramount to our success.

Thank you to our friends James Lincoln (for taking photographs with zero direction) ★, Simon Songhurst ▲ and Elisabeth Hoff ♦ for all their stunning photographs, without which this book would be rather dull to look at.

Thanks to Danny and Steve at Type & Numbers for designing this book so beautifully.

Thanks to Stacey for helping us with this book and being the best friend anyone could ask for. May the Armchair Detectives live on forever!

Thank you to Amy for eating all the biscuits, chocolates, marshmallows, cake pops, macaroons and sweets that come with the daily Pixiwoo post, so that we don't have to. We'll pay for your dental bills when your teeth fall out!

Pixiwoo